SLIM & STRONG:

Quick and Easy Weight Loss Tips for Women.

Achieve Your Dream Body with Simple, Effective Strategies for Fast Results

SAM ABABIO

DEDICATION

To my family, whose unwavering support and love have been my foundation,

To my friends, who have inspired and encouraged me every step of the way,

And to all the dreamers and doers, who strive for success and never give up,

This book is dedicated to you.

May it be a guide and a source of inspiration on your journey to achieving your dreams.

With heartfelt gratitude.

TABLE OF CONTENT

DEDICATION 3

Introduction: Your Path to Slim & Strong 5

Chapter 1: Understanding Your Body's Needs...................10

Chapter 2: The Power of Simple, Balanced Eating............16

Conclusion: The Power of Simple, Balanced Eating 22

Chapter 3: Quick Workouts for Maximum Impact............23

Conclusion: Quick Workouts, Lasting Results 30

Chapter 4: Healthy Habits That Stick 31

Chapter 5: Overcoming Plateaus and Staying Motivated ..36

Chapter 6: Quick Fixes vs. Sustainable Solutions 41

Chapter 7: The Emotional Side of Weight Loss 47

Conclusion: Nurturing Your Emotional Well-Being on the Journey to Slim & Strong 52

Chapter 8: Success Stories: Real Women, Real Results 53

Conclusion: Your Slim & Strong Journey...........................58

Introduction: Your Path to Slim & Strong

Embarking on a journey to achieve weight loss can be both empowering and challenging, especially for women who often face unique obstacles that require a nuanced approach. This introduction lays the foundation for what you can expect from Slim & Strong: Quick and Easy Weight Loss Tips for Women. We'll address the specific weight loss challenges women encounter, debunk common myths, and highlight the importance of a balanced approach that is both quick and sustainable.

Overview of Weight Loss Challenges Specific to Women

Weight loss is a highly individualized process, and for women, it can be particularly complex due to biological, psychological, and social factors. Here's a breakdown of some of the key challenges women face:

1. **Hormonal Fluctuations**: Women experience regular hormonal shifts throughout their lives—during menstruation, pregnancy, postpartum, and menopause—that can affect metabolism, fat storage, and energy levels. For example, during the menstrual cycle, estrogen and progesterone levels fluctuate, leading to water retention, cravings, and changes in appetite, making it harder to stick to a diet or workout routine.

   Menopause presents an even greater challenge as it often leads to a slower metabolism, making it easier to gain weight, especially around the midsection. Additionally, declining estrogen levels can lead to a reduction in muscle mass, which further impacts metabolic rate and fat-burning capacity.

2. **Metabolic Differences**: On average, women have a lower basal metabolic rate (BMR) compared to men, meaning they burn fewer calories at rest. This difference is partly due to higher body fat percentages and lower muscle mass in women. Muscle mass plays a critical role in calorie burning, so lower levels in women can make it harder to lose weight quickly.

3. **Psychological and Emotional Factors**: Women are more likely to experience emotional eating, often turning to food as a coping mechanism for stress, sadness, or anxiety. This can sabotage even the most well-intentioned weight loss efforts. Additionally, women often face societal pressure to look a certain way, which can lead to unhealthy dieting behaviors or a focus on rapid, unsustainable weight loss.

4. **Social Expectations and Time Constraints**: Many women balance multiple roles as caregivers, professionals, and partners. This can leave little time for self-care, including exercise and meal prep. The demands of daily life can make it difficult to prioritize fitness and healthy eating, leading to reliance on convenient but unhealthy food options.

Debunking Common Myths and Misconceptions About Losing Weight

There is no shortage of misinformation when it comes to weight loss, and women are often the target of fad diets, unrealistic promises, and quick-fix solutions that fail to deliver long-term results. Let's clear up some of the most common myths:

1. **Myth: Starving Yourself Is the Fastest Way to Lose Weight**: Many women believe that eating as little as possible is the quickest route to weight loss. However, drastically cutting calories can backfire. When you eat too little, your body goes into "starvation mode," slowing down your metabolism to conserve energy. This makes it harder to lose weight and easier to regain it once you start eating normally again. Instead, a balanced, calorie-controlled diet that includes nutrient-dense foods is the key to sustainable weight loss.

2. **Myth: Carbs Are the Enemy**: Low-carb diets have been popularized in recent years, but the idea that all carbohydrates are bad for weight loss is misleading. Carbohydrates provide energy, and the body needs them to fuel physical activity. The key is to focus on the right types of carbs—complex carbohydrates like whole grains, fruits, and vegetables—rather than refined carbs such as white bread and sugary snacks. These healthier carbs provide essential nutrients and keep you fuller for longer.

3. **Myth: Cardio Is the Only Way to Lose Fat**: Many women assume that endless hours of cardio are the best way to burn fat. While cardio exercises like running and cycling are great for heart health and calorie burning, strength training is equally important for fat loss. Building muscle through resistance training increases your metabolic rate, meaning you burn more calories even at rest. Incorporating both cardio and strength training into your routine is the most effective approach.

4. **Myth: You Can Spot-Reduce Fat**: One of the most persistent myths is that you can lose fat in specific areas by targeting them with exercises, such as doing hundreds of crunches to lose belly fat. In reality, fat loss happens across the body as a whole, not in isolated spots. A well-rounded fitness plan that combines cardio, strength training, and flexibility exercises will help you reduce overall body fat and improve muscle tone.

The Importance of a Balanced Approach: Quick, but Sustainable

When it comes to weight loss, many women seek fast results, but quick fixes can often lead to disappointment, frustration, and even weight gain in the long run. The key to successful weight loss is striking a balance between achieving quick progress and ensuring that the changes you make are sustainable over time. Here's why a balanced approach matters:

1. **Focusing on Long-Term Success**: Extreme diets and workout plans may provide rapid results, but they are rarely sustainable. Overly restrictive eating and intense exercise regimens can lead to burnout, making it difficult to maintain weight loss. Instead, adopting a balanced approach that allows for flexibility and gradual progress sets you up for long-term success. The goal is to create healthy habits you can stick to for life, not just for a few weeks.

2. **Maintaining Muscle Mass**: Quick weight loss often comes at the expense of muscle mass, especially when the focus is solely on calorie

restriction or excessive cardio. Preserving muscle mass is crucial for a healthy metabolism. By incorporating strength training and eating adequate protein, you can ensure that your body burns fat while maintaining lean muscle, which will help you stay strong and toned as you lose weight.

3. **Promoting Overall Health**: Rapid weight loss methods, such as crash diets, can lead to nutritional deficiencies and harm your overall health. A balanced approach prioritizes nutrient-dense foods that provide your body with the vitamins, minerals, and macronutrients it needs to function properly. This not only supports weight loss but also boosts energy, improves mood, and enhances overall well-being.

4. **Preventing Weight Regain**: One of the biggest challenges with fast weight loss is keeping the weight off. Studies show that individuals who lose weight quickly are more likely to regain it over time. A gradual, balanced approach allows your body to adjust to the changes, making it easier to maintain your new weight. By developing healthy habits—like regular exercise, portion control, and mindful eating—you set yourself up for lasting success.

Chapter 1: Understanding Your Body's Needs

Achieving sustainable weight loss requires a deep understanding of how your body works, especially as a woman. The female body has unique physiological and hormonal factors that can affect how it burns calories, stores fat, and builds muscle. This chapter dives into the science of female metabolism, the hormonal factors influencing weight loss, and how to tailor your weight loss approach to your age, lifestyle, and specific goals.

The Science of Female Metabolism

Metabolism refers to the chemical processes in your body that convert food into energy. Your metabolic rate is the speed at which your body burns calories to fuel everything from basic functions (breathing, circulating blood) to more strenuous activities like exercising. Several factors affect a woman's metabolic rate, including age, muscle mass, and activity levels. Understanding these factors can help you make more informed choices when trying to lose weight.

1. **Basal Metabolic Rate (BMR)**: Basal metabolic rate (BMR) is the number of calories your body needs to perform basic life-sustaining functions at rest. Women generally have a lower BMR than men due to physiological differences such as having less muscle mass and more body fat. Since muscle is more metabolically active than fat, women tend to burn fewer calories at rest. This means that while women may require fewer calories, building and maintaining muscle mass is crucial for boosting metabolism and supporting fat loss.

- o **How to Boost BMR**: Incorporating strength training into your routine is one of the most effective ways to increase muscle mass, which in turn elevates your BMR. Additionally, eating enough protein helps preserve muscle tissue during weight loss, preventing your body from burning muscle for energy.

2. **Thermic Effect of Food (TEF)**: The thermic effect of food (TEF) refers to the calories your body uses to digest, absorb, and process food. Certain foods, like protein-rich foods, require more energy to digest than carbohydrates and fats. While TEF plays a smaller role in total calorie expenditure compared to BMR, it highlights the importance of food quality. Choosing nutrient-dense, high-protein foods can give your metabolism a slight boost while helping you stay full and satisfied.

3. **Non-Exercise Activity Thermogenesis (NEAT)**: NEAT accounts for the calories burned during daily activities like walking, standing, and even fidgeting. Women with busy, active lifestyles tend to have higher NEAT levels, contributing significantly to overall calorie expenditure. Incorporating more movement into your day, even if it's not structured exercise, can increase your daily calorie burn and support weight loss.

Hormonal Factors Affecting Weight Loss

Hormones play a critical role in regulating metabolism, appetite, and fat storage, and their influence on weight loss is particularly significant for women. Throughout different life stages, hormonal fluctuations can either support or hinder weight loss efforts. Here are the key hormones that impact women's ability to lose weight:

1. **Estrogen**: Estrogen is the primary female sex hormone, and it fluctuates throughout a woman's life—from puberty to menopause. In terms of weight loss, estrogen helps regulate fat storage, particularly in the lower body (hips, thighs, and buttocks). While higher estrogen levels tend to promote fat storage, especially during childbearing years, lower estrogen levels, such as during menopause, can shift fat storage to the abdominal area and make it harder to lose weight. This is why many women experience weight gain around the midsection as they age.

   o **Managing Estrogen Imbalances**: Maintaining a balanced diet, managing stress, and staying active can help regulate estrogen levels. Foods like cruciferous vegetables (broccoli, kale) may also support estrogen metabolism. Strength training is particularly beneficial for women approaching menopause, as it helps counteract the loss of muscle mass and increases calorie burning.

2. **Progesterone**: Progesterone, another key hormone in the menstrual cycle, works in balance with estrogen. It tends to cause water retention and bloating, particularly during the luteal phase (the second half of the menstrual cycle), which can make you feel heavier and may mask fat loss progress. While it doesn't directly contribute to fat gain, the discomfort associated with water retention can lead to emotional eating or a lack of motivation to exercise.

   o **Dealing with Water Retention**: Staying hydrated, reducing sodium intake, and engaging in light exercise during the luteal phase can help minimize bloating and water retention. Monitoring your weight over time, rather than daily, can also prevent discouragement caused by temporary fluctuations.

3. **Cortisol**: Cortisol is known as the "stress hormone" and is released in response to stress. Chronic stress leads to elevated cortisol levels, which can increase appetite, particularly for high-fat, sugary foods, and promote fat storage, especially in the abdominal area. High cortisol levels also interfere with sleep, which further disrupts metabolism and can lead to weight gain.
   - **Lowering Cortisol Levels**: Stress management is crucial for successful weight loss. Practices such as meditation, yoga, and deep breathing can help reduce cortisol levels. Ensuring you get enough sleep each night also plays a vital role in regulating cortisol and supporting weight loss.

4. **Insulin**: Insulin is responsible for regulating blood sugar levels. When you eat carbohydrates, your body releases insulin to help shuttle glucose (sugar) into your cells for energy. However, chronic overeating or eating too many refined carbs can lead to insulin resistance, where your body becomes less effective at using insulin. This can lead to excess fat storage, particularly around the belly.
   - **Improving Insulin Sensitivity**: Reducing your intake of processed carbs and sugars, increasing fiber-rich foods, and exercising regularly (especially strength training and HIIT workouts) can improve insulin sensitivity and help your body burn fat more effectively.

Tailoring Your Approach to Your Age, Lifestyle, and Goals

No two women are the same, and your weight loss strategy should reflect your unique circumstances. Tailoring your approach to your age, lifestyle, and specific goals is critical to achieving success in a healthy and sustainable way.

1. **Age-Specific Approaches**:
    - **In Your 20s and 30s**: During these years, many women have a higher metabolism and greater muscle mass, making it easier to lose weight. However, stress from career pressures or starting a family can disrupt healthy habits. Focusing on portion control, regular exercise, and managing stress through self-care practices can prevent weight gain and promote long-term health.
    - **In Your 40s and 50s**: As you approach menopause, hormonal changes slow metabolism and reduce muscle mass. Women in this age group should prioritize strength training to preserve muscle, along with a balanced diet rich in lean protein, healthy fats, and fiber. Addressing sleep quality and managing stress become even more important for keeping weight under control.
    - **In Your 60s and Beyond**: Post-menopause, the focus should shift to maintaining mobility, bone health, and preventing further muscle loss. Low-impact exercises such as walking, swimming, and yoga, combined with strength training, can help keep the body strong. Diet should focus on nutrient-dense foods, and attention should be given to portion sizes as metabolism naturally slows with age.

2. **Lifestyle Considerations**: Your daily routine, work environment, and family obligations all impact how you approach weight loss. For busy women, finding quick and effective ways to incorporate movement is crucial, whether it's walking during lunch breaks or doing short home workouts. If you have limited time, focusing on high-intensity interval training (HIIT) and strength training can maximize results in less time.

   - **Finding a Sustainable Routine**: Tailoring your fitness plan to fit your lifestyle ensures consistency. If you have young children, for example, incorporating family-friendly physical activities like biking or hiking can help you stay active. Likewise, meal planning and prepping in advance can help you avoid unhealthy eating patterns during busy work weeks.

3. **Setting Realistic Goals**: Weight loss goals should be specific, measurable, and realistic. Rather than focusing solely on the number on the scale, consider other markers of success, such as improved energy levels, better sleep, and increased strength. Losing 1-2 pounds per week is considered a healthy rate of weight loss, and setting short-term goals that build toward your long-term vision will help keep you motivated.

   - **Tracking Progress**: Keeping a journal of your food intake, exercise, and how you feel can provide valuable insights into what's working and what needs adjustment. Celebrating non-scale victories, such as fitting into your clothes better or having more stamina, can keep you focused on the bigger picture.

Chapter 2: The Power of Simple, Balanced Eating

Diet plays an essential role in achieving lasting weight loss, but it doesn't have to be overly complex or restrictive. In fact, one of the most powerful strategies for weight loss is mastering the basics: portion control, balanced meals, and mindful eating. In this chapter, we'll explore easy-to-follow guidelines that demystify healthy eating and show how small, consistent changes can lead to significant results.

Easy-to-Follow Guidelines for Portion Control

Portion control is one of the most effective ways to manage calorie intake without feeling deprived. The goal isn't to eat less but to eat the right amounts of food, tailored to your body's needs. Here are a few practical tips to help you master portion control:

1. **Visual Cues for Portion Sizes**: One of the easiest ways to manage portion sizes is by using visual references instead of obsessing over calorie counting. For example:
   - A portion of protein (chicken, fish, or tofu) should be about the size of your palm.
   - A serving of carbohydrates (rice, pasta, or potatoes) should be around the size of a clenched fist.
   - Healthy fats (olive oil, nuts, or avocado) can be measured by a thumb-sized amount.
   - A portion of vegetables should fill at least half of your plate.
2. **Plate Method for Balanced Meals**: The plate method is a simple and effective way to create

balanced meals. Visualize your plate divided into sections:

- o **Half of the plate** should consist of non-starchy vegetables (e.g., leafy greens, broccoli, bell peppers).
- o **One quarter** should be lean protein (e.g., chicken, fish, beans).
- o **One quarter** should be whole grains or starchy vegetables (e.g., quinoa, sweet potatoes).

This method not only helps control portions but also ensures you're getting a balance of nutrients at every meal.

3. **Avoiding Portion Creep**: Over time, it's easy to lose sight of portion sizes, leading to gradual overeating. One way to combat this is by eating off smaller plates and bowls, which naturally reduces the amount of food you serve yourself. Additionally, practicing mindful eating (discussed later in the chapter) can help you tune into hunger and fullness cues, preventing overeating.

Meal Timing and the Benefits of Mindful Eating

While what you eat matters, when and how you eat can also influence your weight loss success. Meal timing and mindful eating are two strategies that can enhance your eating habits and prevent overeating.

1. **Meal Timing**: Eating at regular intervals throughout the day helps stabilize blood sugar levels and prevents extreme hunger, which can lead

to overeating. Here are some guidelines for meal timing:

- o **Breakfast**: Kickstart your metabolism with a balanced breakfast within an hour of waking up. Including protein (e.g., eggs, yogurt, or protein shakes) helps keep you full until your next meal.
- o **Snacks**: If you tend to get hungry between meals, plan for healthy snacks like nuts, fruits, or vegetables with hummus to prevent overeating at your next meal.
- o **Dinner**: Try to have your last meal of the day at least 2-3 hours before bedtime to aid digestion and support a good night's sleep.

There is no universal "best" meal timing strategy, but consistency is key. Eating meals at roughly the same time each day helps regulate your appetite and supports long-term weight loss.

2. **Mindful Eating**: Mindful eating is the practice of being fully present during your meals—focusing on the taste, texture, and smell of your food while paying attention to hunger and fullness cues. This practice not only enhances your enjoyment of food but can also help prevent overeating and promote better digestion.

Some ways to practice mindful eating include:

- o **Eating without distractions**: Avoid eating in front of the TV or while scrolling through your phone. By eliminating distractions, you can focus on the act of eating and recognize when you're truly full.
- o **Chewing slowly**: Slowing down the pace of your meals gives your brain time to catch up with

> your stomach's fullness signals. Aim to chew each bite thoroughly and savor the flavors of your food.
>
> - o **Listening to your body**: Practice tuning in to your hunger and fullness signals. Eat when you're genuinely hungry, and stop eating when you feel satisfied—not stuffed.

How to Create Quick, Nutritious Meals with Minimal Effort

Busy lifestyles often make it challenging to cook healthy meals from scratch every day. However, with some planning and smart choices, you can create quick, nutritious meals with minimal effort. Here are some practical strategies for simplifying meal prep:

1. **Meal Prepping in Batches**: Batch cooking is an excellent way to ensure you have healthy meals ready throughout the week. Set aside a few hours once a week to cook large portions of staple ingredients (e.g., grilled chicken, roasted vegetables, quinoa) that can be mixed and matched for various meals. Store these in portioned containers so you can grab them quickly during the week.

2. **One-Pan or Sheet-Pan Meals**: One-pan or sheet-pan meals are lifesavers when you want minimal cleanup. Simply arrange protein (like chicken or salmon) and vegetables on a baking sheet, drizzle with olive oil, sprinkle your favorite seasonings, and roast everything together. In about 30 minutes, you'll have a complete meal with little fuss.

3. **Make Use of Frozen and Canned Foods**: Don't underestimate the convenience and nutrition of frozen and canned foods. Frozen vegetables, fruits, and lean proteins like fish can be just as nutritious as fresh options and are ready to use without much prep. Canned beans, chickpeas, and tomatoes are also great pantry staples for quick meals.

4. **Healthy Convenience Foods**: While fresh, homemade meals are ideal, there are many healthy convenience foods that can save time without sacrificing nutrition. Pre-washed salads, rotisserie chicken, and pre-cut vegetables are excellent shortcuts when you're in a rush. Pair these with whole grains or healthy fats for a balanced, satisfying meal.

Bonus: Sample Meal Plans and Grocery Lists

To help you put these strategies into action, here are some sample meal plans and grocery lists that incorporate the principles of balanced eating, portion control, and mindful meal prep.

Sample Meal Plan #1 (Busy Weekday Routine):

- **Breakfast**: Greek yogurt with mixed berries and a sprinkle of nuts.
- **Lunch**: Quinoa salad with roasted vegetables, chickpeas, and a lemon-tahini dressing.
- **Snack**: Apple slices with almond butter.
- **Dinner**: Sheet-pan chicken with roasted sweet potatoes and green beans.

- **Dessert (optional)**: A small square of dark chocolate.

Sample Meal Plan #2 (Meal Prep-Friendly):

- **Breakfast**: Overnight oats with chia seeds, almond milk, and fresh berries.
- **Lunch**: Grilled chicken with brown rice and steamed broccoli (batch cooked).
- **Snack**: Carrot sticks with hummus.
- **Dinner**: Stir-fry with tofu, mixed vegetables, and whole grain noodles (batch cooked).
- **Dessert (optional)**: Greek yogurt with a drizzle of honey.

Grocery List:

- Lean proteins: chicken breasts, salmon, tofu, Greek yogurt
- Whole grains: quinoa, brown rice, oats
- Vegetables: spinach, broccoli, carrots, green beans, bell peppers
- Fruits: berries, apples, bananas
- Healthy fats: olive oil, nuts, avocado
- Snacks: hummus, almond butter, dark chocolate

Conclusion: The Power of Simple, Balanced Eating

Eating for weight loss doesn't have to be complicated or stressful. By focusing on portion control, mindful eating, and easy meal planning, you can fuel your body in a way that supports both quick results and long-term success. The key is consistency—small, simple changes made over time will lead to lasting transformation, helping you become Slim & Strong without sacrificing your enjoyment of food.

Chapter 3: Quick Workouts for Maximum Impact

Time is one of the biggest challenges women face when it comes to staying fit. Between work, family, and social obligations, finding the time to exercise can feel impossible. The good news is, you don't need hours at the gym to see results. Short, effective workouts—done consistently—can have a powerful impact on your fitness, strength, and weight loss goals. This chapter explores the importance of strength training and cardio, provides 15-minute fat-burning workouts, and shows you how to incorporate movement into your busy lifestyle with illustrated routines that target key areas like arms, core, and legs.

The Importance of Strength Training and Cardio for Women

When it comes to weight loss and overall fitness, a combination of strength training and cardiovascular exercise is key. Each type of exercise serves a unique purpose, and together, they create a balanced approach to achieving your fitness goals.

1. **Strength Training for Women**: Many women shy away from strength training, fearing it will make them bulky. However, strength training is one of the most effective ways to burn fat, build lean muscle, and reshape your body. The more muscle you have, the more calories your body burns at rest, leading to faster fat loss.

Strength training also has other benefits:

- o **Boosts metabolism**: Muscle tissue burns more calories than fat, even when you're not working out.
- o **Improves bone density**: As women age, they are at higher risk of osteoporosis. Strength training helps protect bones and improves long-term health.
- o **Increases functional strength**: Strength training not only tones your muscles but also makes daily tasks like lifting groceries or carrying kids easier.

2. **Cardiovascular Exercise**: Cardio is essential for burning calories, improving heart health, and boosting stamina. While long cardio sessions can be effective, studies show that short bursts of high-intensity exercise (like HIIT—High-Intensity Interval Training) can be just as powerful for fat loss and overall fitness.

Benefits of cardiovascular exercise include:

- o **Increased calorie burn**: High-intensity cardio creates an "afterburn" effect, where your body continues burning calories even after the workout is over.
- o **Improved endurance**: Cardio workouts help your heart and lungs work more efficiently, making physical activities feel easier over time.
- o **Mood boost**: Cardio stimulates the release of endorphins, the body's natural "feel-good" hormones, which can reduce stress and improve mental well-being.

15-Minute Fat-Burning Workouts You Can Do Anywhere

For busy women, quick workouts are a game-changer. These 15-minute fat-burning routines are designed to fit into your packed schedule while delivering maximum results. Whether you're at home, in the office, or traveling, you can squeeze in one of these routines for a full-body workout.

1. **Full-Body Fat-Burning Circuit**: This high-intensity circuit combines cardio with strength moves to burn fat while building muscle. Do each move for 45 seconds, with a 15-second rest in between.
   - **Jump Squats**: Start with feet shoulder-width apart, squat down, and explode upward into a jump. Land softly and go straight into the next squat.
   - **Push-Ups**: Keep your body in a straight line from head to toe as you lower down and push up. Modify by dropping to your knees if needed.
   - **Mountain Climbers**: Get into a plank position and alternate driving your knees toward your chest as fast as possible.
   - **Plank with Shoulder Taps**: Hold a plank and tap one shoulder with the opposite hand, alternating sides while keeping your core tight.
   - **Burpees**: Stand tall, squat down, kick your feet back into a plank, do a push-up, jump your feet back in, and jump straight up.

   Repeat the circuit three times for a complete 15-minute workout.

2. **Tabata Training**: Tabata is a form of high-intensity interval training (HIIT) that involves 20

seconds of maximum effort followed by 10 seconds of rest, repeated for 8 rounds (4 minutes total for each exercise). Here's a sample Tabata workout:

- o **Jumping Jacks**: 20 seconds on, 10 seconds rest (8 rounds)
- o **Bodyweight Squats**: 20 seconds on, 10 seconds rest (8 rounds)
- o **Plank Hold**: 20 seconds on, 10 seconds rest (8 rounds)

Complete all exercises for a quick but effective 12-minute workout.

3. **Low-Impact Cardio Workout**: For those who want a fat-burning workout without the jumping or high impact, this low-impact cardio routine is perfect.

- o **March in Place**: Lift your knees high and swing your arms to get your heart rate up.
- o **Step-Out Squats**: Step to the side, squat, and step back to the center, alternating sides.
- o **Modified Burpees**: Step back into a plank instead of jumping, then step forward and stand up.
- o **Knee Drives**: Stand with one foot back, drive the knee toward your chest and extend the arms overhead, then switch sides.

Repeat the routine for a total of 15 minutes.

How to Incorporate Movement into a Busy Lifestyle

Exercise doesn't have to come from structured workouts alone. There are countless ways to incorporate movement

into your daily routine, even if you have a busy schedule.
Here are some ideas to help you stay active:

1. **Sneak in Activity Throughout the Day**:
   - **Take the stairs**: Skip the elevator and take the stairs whenever possible.
   - **Walk more**: Park farther away from your destination or take a brisk walk during your lunch break.
   - **Desk workouts**: Do seated leg lifts, calf raises, or shoulder shrugs while sitting at your desk.
   - **Stretch during TV time**: Instead of sitting still while watching TV, use commercial breaks to stretch, do squats, or plank holds.
2. **Set Movement Reminders**: If you're working at a desk or sitting for long periods, set an alarm or reminder to stand up, stretch, or take a short walk every 30-60 minutes. These movement breaks not only burn calories but also improve circulation and reduce stiffness.
3. **Incorporate Family or Friends**: Get your loved ones involved in your fitness routine. Go for walks or hikes with family, invite a friend to join you for a workout, or play active games with your kids. Exercising with others can be more fun and keep you accountable.

Illustrated Workout Routines to Target Key Areas: Arms, Core, Legs

Here are some illustrated workout routines that target common problem areas for women: the arms, core, and legs. Each routine takes less than 15 minutes and can be done with minimal equipment.

1. **Arms & Shoulders (No Equipment Needed)**:
   - **Tricep Dips**: Sit on the edge of a chair, place your hands beside you, and lower your body down by bending your elbows.
   - **Push-Ups**: Regular or modified, focusing on keeping elbows close to your body.
   - **Arm Circles**: Extend your arms out to the sides and make small circles forward and backward to target the shoulders.
   - **Plank to Push-Up**: Start in a plank, then lower one arm at a time into a push-up position and back to plank.
2. **Core (Engage Your Abs)**:
   - **Plank**: Hold a plank position, keeping your body straight and core engaged.
   - **Bicycle Crunches**: Lie on your back and alternate bringing your elbow toward the opposite knee.
   - **Leg Raises**: Lie flat on your back, lift your legs straight up, then slowly lower them without letting them touch the ground.
   - **Russian Twists**: Sit with your legs bent, lean back slightly, and twist from side to side, touching the floor with your hands.
3. **Legs & Glutes (Strengthen and Tone)**:
   - **Squats**: Focus on depth and form, keeping your weight in your heels.
   - **Lunges**: Alternate stepping forward and lowering into a lunge position, targeting the glutes and thighs.
   - **Glute Bridges**: Lie on your back with knees bent, lift your hips toward the ceiling, and squeeze your glutes at the top.
   - **Side Leg Raises**: Lie on your side and lift your top leg toward the ceiling, engaging your outer thigh and glutes.

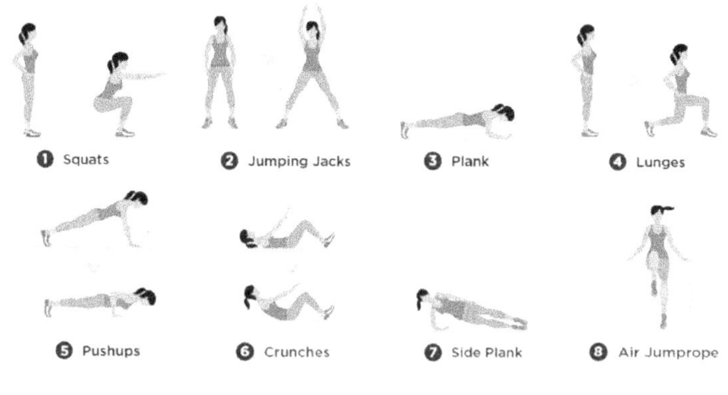

Conclusion: Quick Workouts, Lasting Results

By incorporating these quick, effective workouts into your routine, you'll maximize your results without needing hours in the gym. Whether you have 15 minutes to spare or want to add more movement throughout your day, these strategies will help you build strength, burn fat, and become Slim & Strong. The key is consistency and making fitness a part of your daily lifestyle.

Chapter 4: Healthy Habits That Stick

Losing weight and achieving lasting fitness is more than just about short-term diets or bursts of exercise. Sustainable weight loss comes from building a set of healthy habits that become an integral part of your lifestyle. In this chapter, we'll focus on how to create a daily routine that fosters consistent weight loss, the critical roles that sleep and stress management play in your fitness journey, and small, impactful lifestyle tweaks that can lead to significant long-term results.

Building a Daily Routine for Consistent Weight Loss

A successful weight loss journey depends on the consistency of your daily habits. While big changes can sometimes be overwhelming, it's the smaller, manageable tweaks to your day-to-day routine that will have the most lasting impact. Here are a few essential elements to building a routine that promotes steady, healthy weight loss:

1. **Morning Movement**: Starting your day with some form of physical activity, whether it's a brisk walk, yoga, or strength training, sets the tone for an active and productive day. Even just 10–15 minutes of movement in the morning can kickstart your metabolism, improve your mood, and help you make healthier choices throughout the day.

2. **Meal Prep and Planning**: Preparing meals in advance can make it easier to stick to a healthy eating plan. Take a few hours during the weekend or evenings to cook balanced meals for the week ahead. This prevents impulsive eating and ensures

you always have nutritious options on hand. Having healthy snacks like fruits, nuts, or yogurt easily accessible can also prevent reaching for junk food.

3. **Consistent Meal Timing**: Eating at regular intervals helps regulate your metabolism and prevents overeating. Aim to have meals at roughly the same time each day, and avoid skipping meals, which can lead to overindulgence later. If possible, finish your last meal a few hours before bed to give your body time to digest before sleep.

4. **Track Your Progress**: While weighing yourself daily isn't necessary, keeping a journal or using an app to log meals, exercise, and how you're feeling can help you stay accountable. Tracking habits makes it easier to spot patterns—whether it's a week where you felt particularly energized or one where you may have struggled—and adjust accordingly.

The Role of Sleep and Stress Management in Your Fitness Journey

Two of the most underestimated factors in weight loss and overall health are sleep and stress. Neglecting these two areas can severely impact your progress, even if your diet and exercise routines are on point.

1. **Sleep: The Unsung Hero of Weight Loss**: Poor sleep can derail your fitness goals in several ways. Research shows that people who get less than seven hours of sleep a night are more likely to gain weight. Lack of sleep affects your hunger hormones—ghrelin (which makes you feel hungry) and leptin (which makes you feel full). When you're sleep-deprived, ghrelin levels increase, and leptin

levels drop, making you hungrier and more prone to overeating.

Additionally, being tired leads to poor decision-making, which can lead to choosing unhealthy foods and skipping workouts. Aiming for 7–9 hours of quality sleep each night helps balance your hormones, improve your metabolism, and boost your energy levels for the day ahead.

2. **Stress: The Silent Saboteur**: Chronic stress not only makes it difficult to lose weight but can actually contribute to weight gain, particularly in the abdominal area. When you're stressed, your body produces more cortisol, a hormone that triggers fat storage, especially around the midsection.

    Finding ways to manage stress is crucial for long-term health and weight management. Techniques like meditation, deep breathing exercises, yoga, or even short walks can help reduce stress. Prioritizing activities that bring you joy and relaxation can counteract the negative effects of stress on your body and mind.

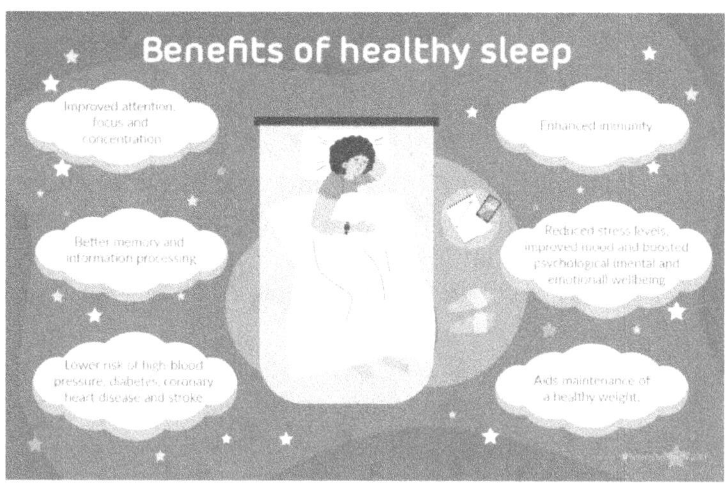

Small Lifestyle Tweaks for Big Results: Hydration, Walking, and More

While diet and exercise are the foundation of weight loss, small lifestyle changes can amplify your results without feeling like a major overhaul. Here are some simple but powerful tweaks you can implement today:

1. **Hydration: Drink More Water**: Drinking enough water is one of the easiest and most effective habits for weight loss. Not only does water help flush out toxins and keep your metabolism running smoothly, but it can also help you feel fuller, preventing overeating. Aiming for 8–10 glasses a day is a good starting point, and drinking a glass of water before meals can help reduce calorie intake. Try replacing sugary drinks or sodas with water or herbal teas to cut down on empty calories.

2. **Walking: The Underrated Fat Burner**: Walking is one of the most accessible forms of exercise and

can significantly contribute to your weight loss goals. Studies show that walking 30 minutes a day can reduce body fat, improve cardiovascular health, and increase stamina. You don't need fancy equipment or a gym membership—just a comfortable pair of shoes. Incorporate more steps into your day by taking the stairs, parking farther away from your destination, or walking during breaks at work.

3. **Eat More Whole Foods**: Whole, unprocessed foods—like vegetables, fruits, lean proteins, whole grains, and healthy fats—are not only nutrient-dense but also more filling, which helps with weight management. Processed foods often contain hidden sugars, unhealthy fats, and empty calories, which can lead to weight gain. By focusing on whole foods, you'll naturally consume fewer calories while nourishing your body with the vitamins and minerals it needs to thrive.

4. **Add Fiber to Your Diet**: Fiber is key to keeping you full, regulating digestion, and aiding in weight loss. Foods high in fiber, such as vegetables, fruits, beans, and whole grains, can help you feel satisfied for longer, preventing overeating. Aim to include fiber-rich foods in every meal to support your weight loss goals.

5. **Create a Support System**: Surrounding yourself with a network of friends, family, or a community with similar health goals can provide motivation and accountability. Joining a workout group, following fitness accounts for inspiration, or even having an accountability partner to check in with can keep you on track.

Chapter 5: Overcoming Plateaus and Staying Motivated

In any weight loss journey, it's common to hit a point where progress slows or even stalls. These moments, known as plateaus, can be frustrating, but they are a natural part of the process. In this chapter, we will explore why plateaus happen and, more importantly, how to break through them. Additionally, we'll cover proven motivation techniques to help you stay on track, the importance of celebrating small victories, and keeping your eyes on long-term goals.

Why Plateaus Happen and How to Break Through Them

Weight loss plateaus occur when your body adapts to your current routine, and what worked initially stops producing the same results. The good news is that plateaus are not a sign of failure but a signal that your body needs a new challenge to continue progressing. Here's a closer look at why plateaus happen and what you can do to overcome them:

1. **Metabolic Adaptation**: As you lose weight, your body requires fewer calories to function. This is a natural biological response; your metabolism slows down as your body adjusts to the lower energy demands. To break through this, you may need to slightly reduce calorie intake or increase physical activity to create a new caloric deficit.
2. **Exercise Routine Stagnation**: If you've been doing the same workout routine for a while, your muscles may no longer be challenged. When your body

becomes efficient at a particular exercise, it burns fewer calories, resulting in slower progress. To overcome this, try switching up your routine by incorporating new exercises, increasing intensity, or adding variety with activities like HIIT (High-Intensity Interval Training) or strength training.

3. **Undereating or Overeating**: It's possible to unknowingly eat too much or too little during your weight loss journey. If you're not consuming enough calories, your body may go into "starvation mode," holding onto fat to preserve energy. Conversely, if you're indulging more than you think, even in healthy foods, you could be unknowingly stalling progress. Tracking your food intake accurately, even for a short time, can help you stay mindful of your diet and make necessary adjustments.

4. **Stress and Sleep Factors**: Stress and poor sleep can significantly impact your weight loss efforts. Both factors can increase cortisol levels, which contribute to fat retention, especially in the abdominal area. Managing stress through mindfulness techniques, regular relaxation, and prioritizing sleep can help you overcome plateaus and regain momentum.

Proven Motivation Techniques to Stay on Track

Staying motivated during a plateau can be difficult, but it's crucial to maintain focus and avoid slipping back into old habits. Here are some techniques to help keep you motivated:

1. **Revisit Your "Why"**: One of the best ways to reignite motivation is to remind yourself why you started your weight loss journey in the first place. Whether it's for health reasons, increased energy, or confidence, reconnecting with your original purpose can provide the emotional boost you need to push forward.

2. **Set New, Short-Term Goals**: If your weight loss progress has stalled, shifting focus to non-scale victories (NSVs) can renew motivation. These can include improving your fitness levels, increasing strength, or fitting into a specific outfit. Setting short-term goals, like completing a certain number of workouts per week or mastering a new exercise, keeps you engaged and provides a sense of accomplishment.

3. **Track Your Progress Beyond the Scale**: Progress isn't only reflected in the number on the scale. Take measurements of your body (waist, hips, arms, etc.) to track changes, or take progress photos every few weeks. Seeing how your body changes visually can be incredibly motivating, even if the scale isn't moving. Remember, muscle weighs more than fat, so while you may not be losing weight, you could be losing inches and toning up.

4. **Create a Vision Board**: A vision board is a visual representation of your goals and aspirations. Fill it with images, quotes, and affirmations that inspire you to stay committed. Display it somewhere visible, and revisit it whenever your motivation dips. It's a fun and creative way to stay focused on the big picture.

5. **Join a Support Group or Fitness Community**: Surrounding yourself with like-minded individuals can provide the encouragement and accountability you need to keep going. Whether it's an online

community, a workout buddy, or joining a local fitness class, sharing your challenges and successes with others makes the journey feel less isolating and more enjoyable.

How to Celebrate Small Wins and Keep Long-Term Goals in Sight

One of the most effective ways to stay motivated is to celebrate small victories along the way. Focusing solely on the end goal can make the process feel long and daunting, but acknowledging progress at each stage makes the journey more rewarding and enjoyable.

1. **Celebrate Milestones**: Weight loss is not just about reaching your final target—it's about progress. Celebrate when you lose your first five or ten pounds, complete a challenging workout, or make a healthy choice when tempted by junk food. These milestones are steps toward your ultimate goal and deserve recognition. Reward yourself with non-food-related treats, like a new workout outfit, a massage, or a day off to relax.

2. **Practice Gratitude for Your Body**: Rather than focusing on what you still need to accomplish, take time to appreciate what your body has already achieved. Celebrate its strength, endurance, and resilience. Practicing body positivity can help shift your mindset from frustration to gratitude, keeping you motivated to continue improving your health.

3. **Break Your Big Goal into Smaller Steps**: If your goal is to lose 30 pounds, that can feel overwhelming. Instead, break it down into smaller, more manageable goals, like losing five pounds at a

time. Focus on incremental changes, and each time you achieve one of these mini-goals, it reinforces the idea that you are capable of reaching the larger target.

4. **Keep Your Long-Term Vision in Mind**: While celebrating small wins is important, it's also essential to keep your long-term goals in sight. Use affirmations and visual reminders (like your vision board) to stay connected to your big "why" and the overall transformation you're striving for. Set calendar reminders or journal about how far you've come to maintain perspective.

Chapter 6: Quick Fixes vs. Sustainable Solutions

In the pursuit of weight loss, it's easy to be tempted by promises of quick fixes and fast results. The internet and media are filled with fad diets, miracle pills, and extreme workout plans that claim to transform your body in just a few weeks. While these approaches may yield short-term results, they are often unsustainable, leading to weight regain and even long-term harm to your health. This chapter will explore the differences between quick fixes and sustainable solutions, explain why slow and steady progress is the key to lasting success, and provide strategies for maintaining your healthy lifestyle once you've reached your goal.

How to Avoid Fad Diets and Unhealthy Quick Fixes

Fad diets and extreme solutions have become a common trap for many people looking to lose weight quickly. From restrictive calorie counting to eliminating entire food groups, these diets often promise rapid results but rarely consider the long-term consequences. Here's how to recognize and avoid these unhealthy methods:

1. **Recognizing Fad Diets**: Fad diets usually have a few common characteristics:
    - **Extreme Restrictions**: They often require you to eliminate essential food groups, like carbohydrates or fats, which can lead to nutrient deficiencies.
    - **Promises of Rapid Weight Loss**: Any diet that guarantees losing more than 2 pounds per week

is likely promoting unhealthy, unsustainable habits.

- o **Lack of Scientific Support**: Fad diets are typically not based on credible scientific evidence, and many are debunked by experts in nutrition and health.
- o **Overly Simplistic Rules**: These diets often oversimplify weight loss by claiming that eating or avoiding specific foods will solve all your problems. Examples include the grapefruit diet, cabbage soup diet, or juice cleanses.

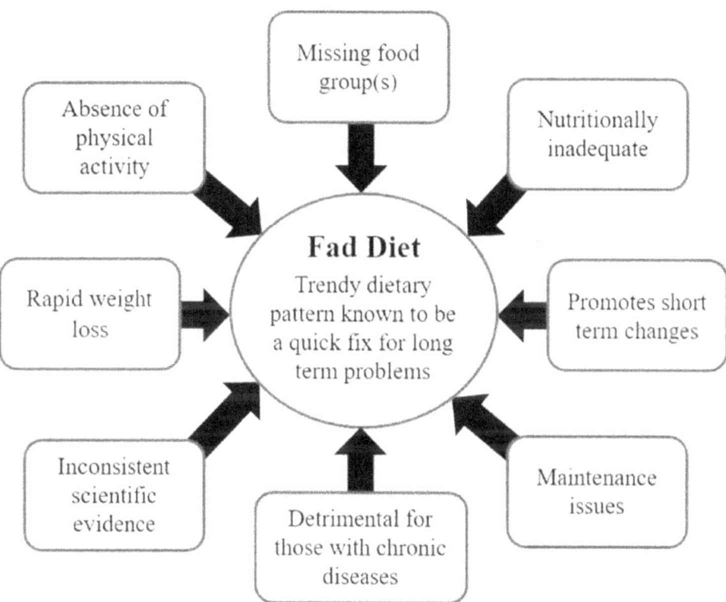

2. **The Dangers of Quick Fixes**: While quick fixes may provide immediate gratification, they often come with hidden costs:

- o **Nutritional Deficiencies**: Diets that cut out major food groups can lead to a lack of essential nutrients, causing fatigue, weakened immunity, and long-term health problems.

- o **Metabolic Damage**: Extreme calorie restriction can slow down your metabolism, making it harder to lose weight in the future.
- o **Yo-Yo Dieting**: Most quick fixes are impossible to maintain over the long term. When you inevitably return to normal eating habits, the weight usually comes back, often leading to a cycle of losing and regaining weight, known as yo-yo dieting.
- o **Mental and Emotional Stress**: Quick fixes can also take a toll on your mental health, leading to stress, anxiety, and an unhealthy relationship with food.

Why Slow, Steady Progress Leads to Lasting Results

Sustainable weight loss is about developing healthy habits that you can maintain for life. Although it may take longer to see results with a balanced approach, the benefits are far more significant in the long run. Here's why slow and steady progress leads to lasting results:

1. **Building Healthy Habits**: Sustainable weight loss is built on a foundation of healthy habits, such as balanced eating, regular exercise, and proper self-care. When you focus on slow progress, you give yourself the time to establish these habits in a way that feels natural and manageable. Over time, these habits become part of your routine, making it easier to maintain your weight loss and overall health.
2. **Preserving Muscle Mass**: Quick fixes often result in rapid weight loss, but much of that loss comes from muscle rather than fat. Losing muscle can slow down your metabolism and make it harder to

keep the weight off. Slow, steady progress, combined with strength training, ensures that you lose fat while preserving lean muscle, which is essential for maintaining a healthy metabolism.

3. **Avoiding the Stress of Extreme Measures**: Fad diets and quick fixes are mentally exhausting. They require constant vigilance and often create feelings of guilt or frustration when you slip up. On the other hand, a slow, steady approach allows for flexibility and enjoyment. You don't have to deprive yourself of your favorite foods or feel like you're constantly on a strict plan. This leads to a healthier relationship with food and less stress overall.

4. **More Sustainable Metabolism**: When you lose weight gradually, your body has time to adjust to the changes. This reduces the risk of metabolic slowdown, where your body burns fewer calories to conserve energy. By focusing on gradual weight loss, you can prevent this from happening and keep your metabolism running efficiently.

5. **Long-Term Psychological Benefits**: Slow and steady weight loss allows you to develop a positive mindset toward your body and the changes you're making. As you see progress over time, you build confidence in your ability to maintain a healthy lifestyle. This sense of empowerment can help you stay motivated and committed to your goals for the long term.

Strategies for Maintaining Your New Healthy Lifestyle Once the Weight Is Off

Losing weight is only the first part of the journey. The real challenge is maintaining your progress and avoiding the weight regain that often follows rapid weight loss. Here are some strategies to help you stay on track after reaching your goal:

1. **Focus on Maintenance, Not Perfection**: Once you've lost the weight, the goal shifts from losing more to maintaining your progress. It's essential to embrace the idea of balance rather than perfection. Allow yourself occasional treats and indulgences, but keep overall healthy habits in place. Moderation is key.

2. **Continue Practicing Balanced Eating**: Sustainable weight loss maintenance is built on a diet that is flexible, balanced, and enjoyable. Keep following the principles of portion control, mindful eating, and balanced nutrition that helped you lose weight in the first place. Incorporate a variety of foods from all food groups to ensure you're getting the nutrients you need.

3. **Stay Active**: Regular physical activity is crucial for maintaining your weight. Incorporate movement into your daily routine, whether it's structured exercise like gym workouts or casual activities like walking, dancing, or gardening. Consistency is more important than intensity, so find activities you enjoy and can stick with long-term.

4. **Monitor Your Progress**: While you don't need to weigh yourself every day, regularly checking in with your progress can help you stay accountable. You can monitor your weight, take measurements, or use other indicators like how your clothes fit to

ensure you're maintaining your results. If you notice small fluctuations, adjust your eating and exercise habits before they become bigger problems.

5. **Manage Stress and Get Adequate Sleep**: Stress and lack of sleep can sabotage your efforts by increasing cravings for unhealthy foods and disrupting your hormones. Practice stress management techniques like meditation, deep breathing, or yoga, and prioritize getting at least 7-8 hours of sleep each night. Maintaining a healthy lifestyle is easier when your body and mind are well-rested and calm.

6. **Set New Goals**: Once you've achieved your weight loss goal, it's essential to keep yourself motivated by setting new goals. These goals don't necessarily have to be about weight—they could focus on improving fitness, gaining strength, or adopting a new hobby. By keeping yourself challenged and engaged, you'll be more likely to stick with your healthy habits.

7. **Find a Support System**: Surround yourself with people who support your healthy lifestyle. Whether it's friends, family, or a fitness group, having a community of like-minded individuals can help keep you accountable and motivated. If you find yourself slipping, reach out to your support system for encouragement and guidance.

Chapter 7: The Emotional Side of Weight Loss

Weight loss isn't just a physical journey—it's deeply emotional as well. Many women find that as they shed pounds, they're also confronted with complex feelings about their bodies, self-worth, and societal expectations. In this chapter, we'll explore the connection between mindset and physical transformation, the importance of building body confidence at every stage, and practical strategies for handling self-doubt, emotional eating, and the pressures placed on women by society.

The Connection Between Mindset and Physical Transformation

When embarking on a weight loss journey, it's easy to focus solely on the physical aspects: exercise, diet, and the numbers on the scale. However, your mindset plays a pivotal role in whether or not you'll succeed. Studies show that individuals with a positive, resilient attitude are more likely to maintain healthy habits and achieve long-term results. Here's how mindset influences your weight loss:

1. **The Power of Positive Thinking**:
    - A positive mindset helps you view challenges as opportunities for growth. Instead of becoming discouraged by setbacks, you're more likely to push forward and find solutions.
    - Visualizing your goals and celebrating small victories along the way can reinforce the belief that your transformation is possible, which motivates continued effort.
2. **Building Resilience**:

o   Weight loss doesn't happen overnight, and it's often accompanied by plateaus and setbacks. A resilient mindset enables you to bounce back from these challenges instead of giving up when the process becomes difficult.
o   Cultivating resilience involves recognizing that mistakes are part of the journey and learning to forgive yourself when you slip up. Resilient people focus on progress, not perfection.

3. **Self-Compassion as a Weight Loss Tool**:
o   Many women are their harshest critics, especially when it comes to body image and weight loss. Developing self-compassion means treating yourself with kindness, even when you don't meet your own expectations.
o   Self-compassion helps to break the cycle of negative self-talk and promotes emotional healing, which can reduce stress and emotional eating.

How to Build Body Confidence at Every Stage

Body confidence isn't something that suddenly appears when you reach your goal weight—it's a practice that you can develop at every stage of your weight loss journey. Here's how to cultivate body confidence and embrace your progress:

1. **Appreciating Your Body for What It Can Do**:
o   Shift your focus from how your body looks to what it's capable of. Whether it's completing a challenging workout, walking up the stairs without getting winded, or playing with your kids, recognizing these achievements can foster

a deep sense of gratitude for your body's abilities.

2. **Celebrating Non-Scale Victories**:
   - The number on the scale is just one measure of progress. Celebrate other milestones, such as increased energy levels, improved endurance, fitting into clothes more comfortably, or simply feeling healthier. These non-scale victories reinforce the idea that weight loss is about more than just aesthetics.

3. **Creating a Positive Self-Image**:
   - Engage in activities that make you feel good about yourself. Wearing clothes that make you feel confident, practicing good posture, and engaging in regular self-care can elevate your self-esteem, no matter your current weight.

4. **Body Positivity Throughout the Journey**:
   - It's essential to recognize that body confidence isn't dependent on reaching a specific size. Embrace the fact that your body is constantly evolving, and appreciate it at every stage. Adopting a body-positive attitude doesn't mean you're complacent—it means you're valuing yourself throughout your transformation.

Handling Self-Doubt, Emotional Eating, and Societal Pressures

The emotional side of weight loss is often the most challenging to manage. Self-doubt, emotional eating, and societal pressures can derail even the most dedicated efforts. Here's how to navigate these emotional hurdles and stay focused on your goals:

1. **Conquering Self-Doubt**:

o   It's normal to experience self-doubt during a weight loss journey, especially when progress is slow. Negative thoughts like "I'll never lose the weight" or "I'm not strong enough" can creep in and undermine your confidence.

o   Combat self-doubt by reframing these thoughts into more positive, actionable statements. For example, "I'm working hard and making progress" or "I've overcome challenges before, and I can do it again." Surround yourself with a supportive community—whether it's friends, family, or online groups—that reinforces positive thinking.

2. **Understanding and Managing Emotional Eating**:

o   Emotional eating is a common challenge for women on a weight loss journey. It's when you turn to food for comfort during times of stress, sadness, boredom, or anxiety, rather than hunger. The occasional indulgence is normal, but when emotional eating becomes a habit, it can sabotage your progress.

o   To manage emotional eating, it's essential to identify your emotional triggers. Keep a journal of your feelings when you have cravings, and explore non-food ways to cope with those emotions. Strategies might include going for a walk, practicing mindfulness, or talking to a trusted friend. Additionally, maintaining a balanced diet with regular meals can reduce the likelihood of emotional overeating.

3. **Coping with Societal Pressures**:

o   Society often places enormous pressure on women to look a certain way, which can fuel feelings of inadequacy. From unrealistic beauty standards in the media to social comparisons on platforms like Instagram, it's easy to feel like you're not "enough."

- o The key to overcoming societal pressures is learning to separate your worth from your appearance. Acknowledge that your value as a person isn't tied to your weight or size. Focus on your own goals and remember that everyone's journey is different. Surround yourself with positive, body-inclusive messages and filter out toxic media influences.

Mindset Practices for Emotional Resilience

1. **Mindfulness and Meditation**:
   - o Mindfulness can be a powerful tool in managing emotional challenges and improving your relationship with food and your body. Mindful eating encourages you to slow down, savor each bite, and listen to your body's hunger cues. Meditation can help reduce stress, making you less likely to turn to food for comfort.
2. **Affirmations and Visualization**:
   - o Positive affirmations, such as "I am strong" or "I am capable of reaching my goals," can help shift your mindset and keep you focused. Visualization, where you imagine yourself successfully completing your weight loss journey, can also be a motivating tool.
3. **Journaling**:
   - o Journaling can be a therapeutic outlet for processing emotions and setting intentions. Writing down your thoughts, challenges, and progress can help you gain insight into your mindset and identify patterns that may be holding you back.

Conclusion: Nurturing Your Emotional Well-Being on the Journey to Slim & Strong

As much as weight loss involves physical changes, it's equally about emotional growth. By understanding the powerful connection between mindset and transformation, building body confidence, and learning to manage the emotional challenges that arise, you can set yourself up for long-term success. Remember, the goal isn't just to lose weight but to cultivate a healthier, more empowered relationship with your body, mind, and well-being.

Chapter 8: Success Stories: Real Women, Real Results

Inspiring Case Studies of Women Who Transformed Their Bodies

Wall Pilates has proven to be an incredibly effective workout regimen for women of all ages and fitness levels. In this chapter, we dive into the real-life success stories of women who used Wall Pilates to achieve remarkable transformations. These women come from diverse backgrounds and fitness experiences, yet they all share one common factor: they achieved their goals through dedication, consistency, and a belief in their ability to transform their bodies.

Case Study 1: Emily – The Busy Mom Emily, a 35-year-old mother of two, struggled to find time for herself after having children. Between managing a household, working part-time, and caring for her young kids, her personal fitness had taken a back seat. She often felt exhausted, lacked energy, and was unhappy with her post-pregnancy body.

After stumbling upon Wall Pilates, Emily realized she could easily incorporate short, effective workouts into her daily routine. She began with beginner-level exercises, focusing on core strength and flexibility. Over the course of six months, she progressed to more advanced routines, combining strength training with cardio-based Pilates movements.

Results: Emily lost 20 pounds, regained her energy, and toned her entire body. Her core strength dramatically improved, which also helped alleviate the back pain she had suffered since her pregnancies. Most importantly, she regained her confidence and became an example of how it's possible to fit fitness into a busy life.

Key Takeaway: Consistency and adaptability are key. Even short workouts, when done regularly, can lead to dramatic improvements in body composition and energy levels.

Case Study 2: Sarah – The Career-Focused Professional
At 29, Sarah was thriving in her career, but her fast-paced job in the tech industry left little room for fitness. With long hours at the office and frequent travel, her exercise routine had been inconsistent for years. Sarah gained weight, lost muscle tone, and felt sluggish both physically and mentally.

When Sarah discovered Wall Pilates, she saw an opportunity to integrate fitness into her busy lifestyle without the need for expensive gym memberships or equipment. Starting with just 20 minutes a day, she quickly realized that the wall-assisted exercises not only improved her strength and flexibility but also helped her manage stress.

Results: Over a period of eight months, Sarah lost 15 pounds, sculpted her legs and arms, and developed a stronger core. Wall Pilates also had a mental impact on Sarah—she felt more centered, less stressed, and better able to focus at work. She credits the mind-body connection of Pilates for helping her stay grounded and productive during the workday.

Key Takeaway: Fitness can improve not just your body but your mental well-being. Consistent Pilates practice helps you manage stress, stay focused, and feel more energized—benefits that extend into your professional life.

Case Study 3: Ana – Overcoming Injury and Rebuilding Strength Ana, a 42-year-old avid runner, was sidelined by a knee injury that required surgery. The recovery process was long and frustrating, and she feared that she would never be able to return to her previous level of fitness. After hearing about Wall Pilates from a physical therapist, she decided to give it a try as part of her rehabilitation process.

The wall provided Ana with the support she needed to gradually rebuild her strength, especially in her legs and core, without putting excessive strain on her joints. As her strength and stability improved, Ana slowly incorporated more advanced movements, ultimately regaining her confidence and physical abilities.

Results: Within a year, Ana not only recovered from her injury but also improved her overall fitness level beyond what it had been before her surgery. She credits Wall Pilates for giving her a safe, low-impact way to rebuild strength in her injured knee while also toning her entire body. Today, she has returned to running but continues to practice Wall Pilates to maintain her strength and flexibility.

Key Takeaway: Wall Pilates is a safe, effective way to recover from injury, allowing you to rebuild strength and mobility at your own pace. It's also a sustainable way to prevent future injuries by enhancing flexibility and muscle balance.

Key Lessons Learned from Their Journeys

Through these inspiring transformations, several important lessons stand out that can be applied to your own Wall Pilates journey:

1. **Start Where You Are:** Each of these women started their fitness journeys at different points—whether recovering from injury, balancing a busy schedule, or starting with little to no fitness background. They prove that you don't need to be in perfect shape to begin Wall Pilates. The key is to start where you are and build gradually.
2. **Consistency is Key:** Regardless of the intensity or length of your workout, consistency will always yield results. These women committed to regular practice, often beginning with just a few minutes a day, and saw significant improvements in strength, flexibility, and weight loss.
3. **Adapt Your Routine:** Each person's body and lifestyle are different, and Wall Pilates offers the flexibility to adapt to your unique needs. Whether you're a busy mom, a professional with limited time, or recovering from an injury, Wall Pilates can be tailored to fit into your life.
4. **Mind-Body Connection:** These women found that Wall Pilates helped not only their bodies but also their minds. The practice allowed them to manage stress, stay focused, and improve mental clarity. The importance of the mind-body connection

cannot be overstated, as it enhances the overall impact of your workouts.

5. **Patience and Progress:** Transformation takes time. None of these success stories happened overnight, but with patience and a focus on progress rather than perfection, they each achieved remarkable results. Trust the process, and remember that every small step brings you closer to your goals.

Encouragement to Begin Your Own Transformation

The success stories of these women are not extraordinary because of who they are; they are extraordinary because they made the decision to prioritize their health, fitness, and well-being. If they can do it, so can you.

Wall Pilates offers a versatile, accessible, and effective approach to fitness that can transform not only your body but also your mindset and overall lifestyle. Whether your goal is weight loss, strength building, or simply feeling more confident in your own skin, the only thing standing between you and your transformation is the decision to start.

So, as you turn the page and begin your Wall Pilates journey, know that you are not alone. Countless women have been where you are—wondering if they can truly make a change—and they have succeeded. Now, it's your turn.

Embrace this opportunity, trust in the process, and watch as Wall Pilates helps you achieve your own transformation. You've got this!

Conclusion: Your Slim & Strong Journey

Recap of Key Strategies for Effective, Quick Weight Loss

As you reflect on your Wall Pilates journey, remember the core principles that will continue to guide you towards lasting results:

1. **Consistency Over Intensity:** Small, consistent efforts will always outweigh sporadic, intense workouts. Even 15-20 minutes a day can make a huge difference over time.
2. **Mind-Body Connection:** Focus on engaging your core, breathing deeply, and being mindful of every movement. This connection enhances the effectiveness of your workouts and improves your overall well-being.
3. **Progressive Overload:** As you advance, keep challenging your body with more resistance and complex movements. This approach will ensure continuous muscle growth, strength, and fat loss.
4. **Cardio-Pilates Fusion:** Combining Pilates with low-impact cardio is a game changer for increasing calorie burn, improving cardiovascular health, and speeding up fat loss.
5. **Nutrition and Hydration:** Fueling your body with whole foods, staying hydrated, and practicing portion control are essential for sustainable weight loss and muscle growth.
6. **Flexibility and Mobility:** Prioritize stretches and mobility exercises to prevent injuries, relieve muscle tension, and maintain long-term flexibility and range of motion.
7. **Personalization and Adaptation:** Customize your Wall Pilates routine based on your fitness level and

goals. Listen to your body and make modifications as needed.

Empowering Words to Start Taking Action Today

You've already taken the first step by learning about Wall Pilates, and now it's time to take action. This journey isn't just about losing weight or building strength—it's about becoming the healthiest, most empowered version of yourself.

Change starts with one decision. Whether you're a beginner just getting started or someone looking to elevate your fitness routine, remember that your transformation begins today. Each workout, no matter how small, is a step closer to the strong, confident, and vibrant person you aspire to be.

Don't wait for the perfect moment. Start now. Your future self will thank you.

Final Thoughts on Maintaining Lifelong Health and Confidence

Wall Pilates isn't just a quick-fix solution; it's a sustainable fitness approach that can become part of your lifestyle. Whether you're at home, traveling, or in a gym, this method is adaptable to your needs and goals.

The true power of Wall Pilates lies in its ability to transform not just your body but your mindset. As you continue to grow stronger physically, you'll also gain confidence, energy, and a renewed sense of purpose in your health and wellness journey.

The results you achieve today will build the foundation for a lifetime of health, strength, and self-assurance. Keep moving forward, stay motivated, and embrace the lifelong benefits that Wall Pilates offers.

Bonus Content:

Printable Daily Planners for Meal Prep and Workouts

To help you stay organized and on track, you'll have access to printable daily planners that make it easier to plan meals, track workouts, and visualize your progress. Use these tools to create structure and ensure you're fueling your body properly while keeping up with your Wall Pilates routine.

Access to Exclusive Video Tutorials for At-Home Exercises

As a special bonus, you'll gain access to over 50 exclusive video tutorials that provide clear demonstrations of all the key Wall Pilates movements covered in this book. These videos allow you to follow along at your own pace and ensure proper form for maximum results.

Quick-Reference Cheat Sheet with the Top 10 Tips from the Book

To make it easy to stay on track, we've compiled a quick-reference cheat sheet featuring the top 10 strategies and tips for success from this book. Keep this guide handy for quick motivation and reminders as you continue your fitness journey.

Your journey to becoming slim, strong, and confident is just beginning. Keep pushing forward, and always remember that you are capable of achieving incredible results.

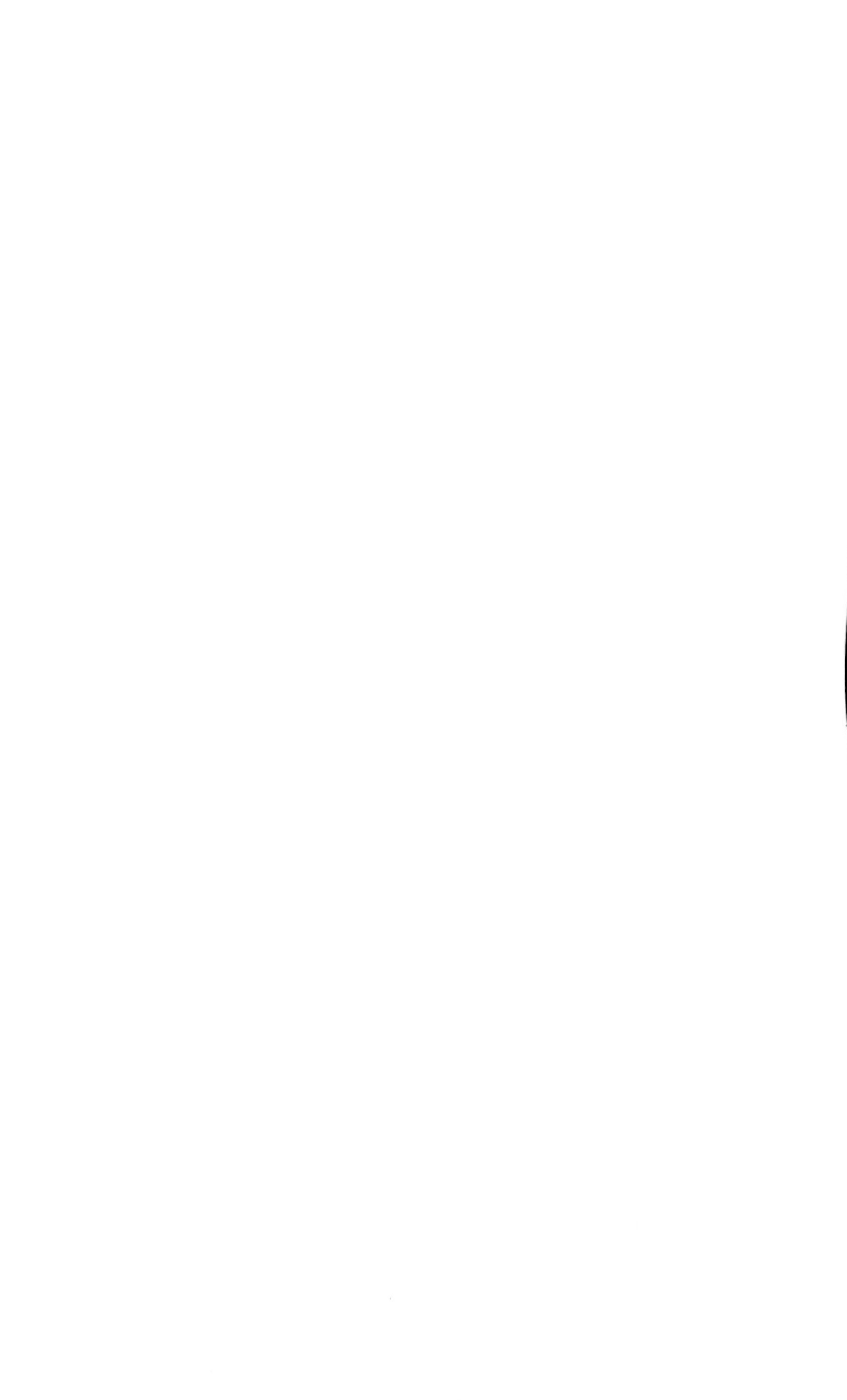